THE STORY OF
PETER PUDGY

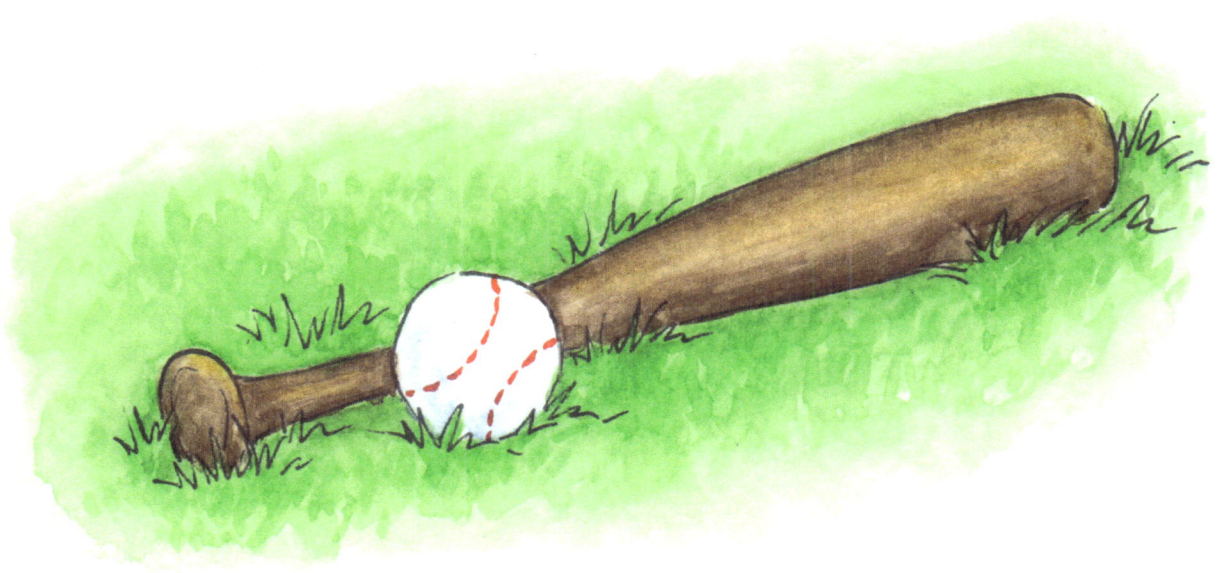

Written by Dr. Maria S. Landis
Edited by Melissa Bailey and Deborah Dyess
Illustrated by Melissa Bailey

Dr. Maria Landis was herself an overweight child. After years of struggling with body image and unkind words, she got fit, and has celebrated her good health ever since. Since 2000, she has been a Personal Trainer, Certified Nutrition Counselor, and Naturopath. Taking a holistic approach to well-being, she enthusiastically shows both children and adults how to create—and maintain—a healthy lifestyle. The school wellness programs she has incorporated into grades K-3 teach students how to choose healthy foods and ways to make exercise fun and invigorating.

Dr. Maria lives in Colorado with her husband Jim and two cats, Samantha and Jasper. In her spare time (*if* she can get any!), she hikes, bikes and fishes in the mountains and is writing her next story.

This is her first children's book.

"Take care of your body.
It's the only place you have to live."

~Jim Rohn

Learn more about Peter's adventure at www.thestoryofpeterpudgy.com.

ACKNOWLEDGEMENTS

What a journey! Along the way, the encouragement from my family and friends gave me the courage and drive to pursue this dream to completion.

Thank you to my editors, Debra Dyess and Melissa Bailey, who brought more life, energy and emotion to the characters and events in this book.

Melissa Bailey is not only an editor but also the illustrator for this story. Each sketch she created became a wonderful creation of the characters and actions in this book. Her expertise in art brings my experience in fitness and nutrition to the world.

Most importantly, my sincere heartfelt appreciation goes to my husband, Jim. Not only did he point out my typos but contributed to the expansion of my ideas and helped keep me focused and encouraged along the way. You are my angel!

Thank you dear Universe for bringing this idea to me!

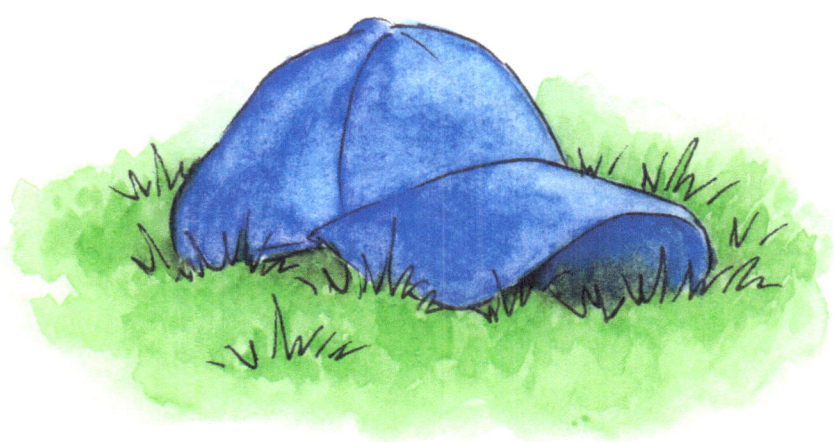

This is the story of how Peter Pudgy changed his name. Peter didn't like being called pudgy, but didn't think he could do anything about it. In fact, he didn't do much of anything at all. He didn't like to run, jump or go outside—and he really didn't even like to walk! But he *did* like food. He ate all day and sat all day. He sat and watched TV and played video games while he ate and ate and ATE.

Peter liked to eat! He also liked baseball, but he wasn't much help to his team, the Good Guys. He was too slow and chubby. But one day, not so long ago, that all changed…

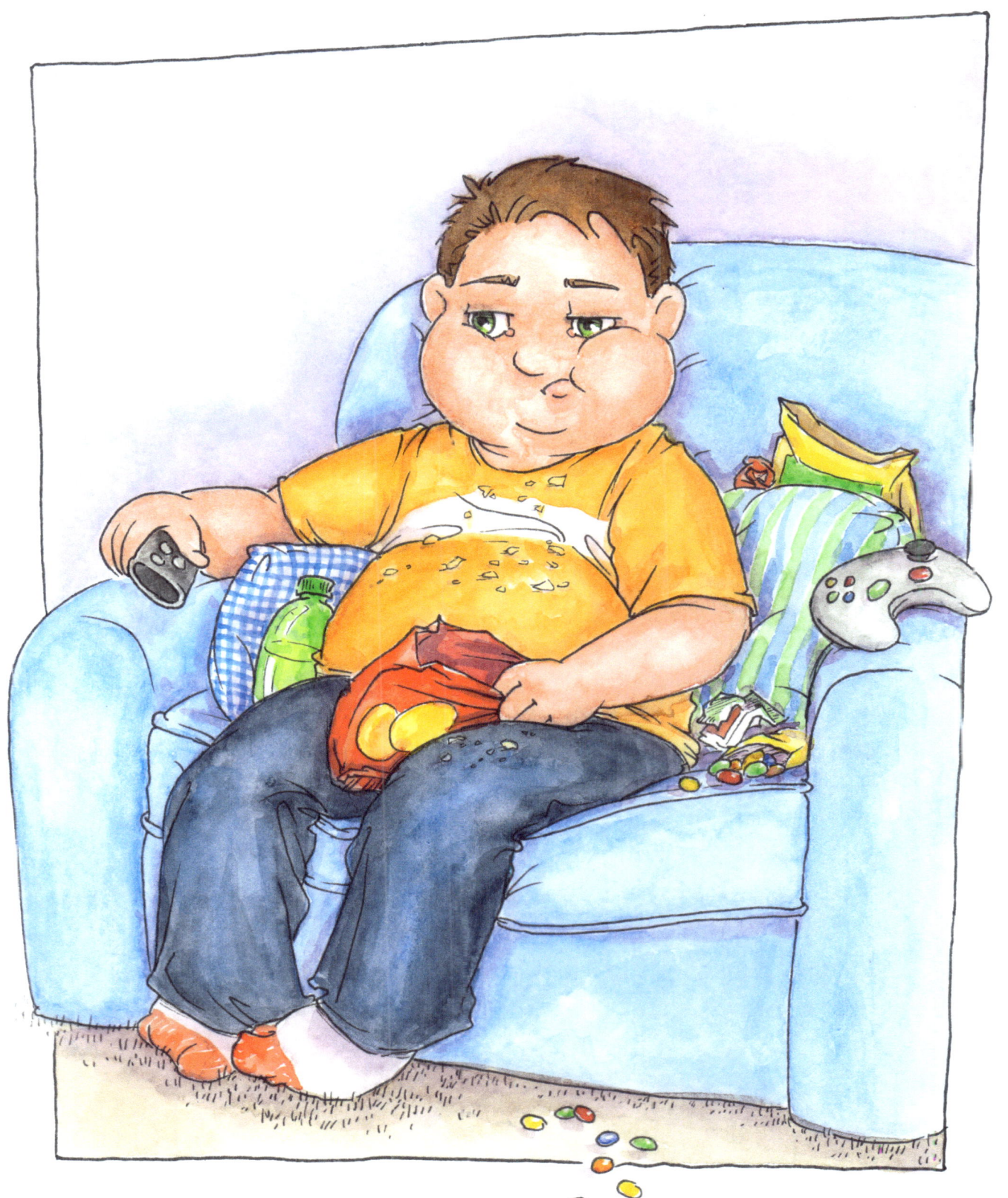

The Good Guys had lost to the Crushers. AGAIN!

Peter looked down at his chubby body with disgust. He wished he looked more like the other boys on his team.

"What are you doing Peter Pudgy?" Tony, the captain of the Crushers, said. He was smirking as he copied Peter trying to make big muscles with his flabby arms. Except Tony's arms were not flabby. His muscles were already big.

Peter thought about telling Tony to stop making fun of him but the last time he tried, Tony tossed him in a garbage can.

"What's the matter Peter Pudgy? Did big, bad Tony hurt your little feelings? Your feelings are the only thing little about you! You take up the whole bench!" Tony laughed, shoved Peter and walked away singing, "Fatty Fatty, two by four; can't get through the dugout door."

Peter sighed. His dream of becoming captain of his baseball team wouldn't ever happen if he looked like *this*.

Peter hated the song Tony made up and didn't like being called Peter Pudgy. Those mean words hurt. Peter wished he could run and play ball without getting out of breath. He tried his best, but sometimes just running to first base made him too tired to play. Then Tony and his buddies would laugh and point at him because he couldn't finish an entire game. It made him sad.

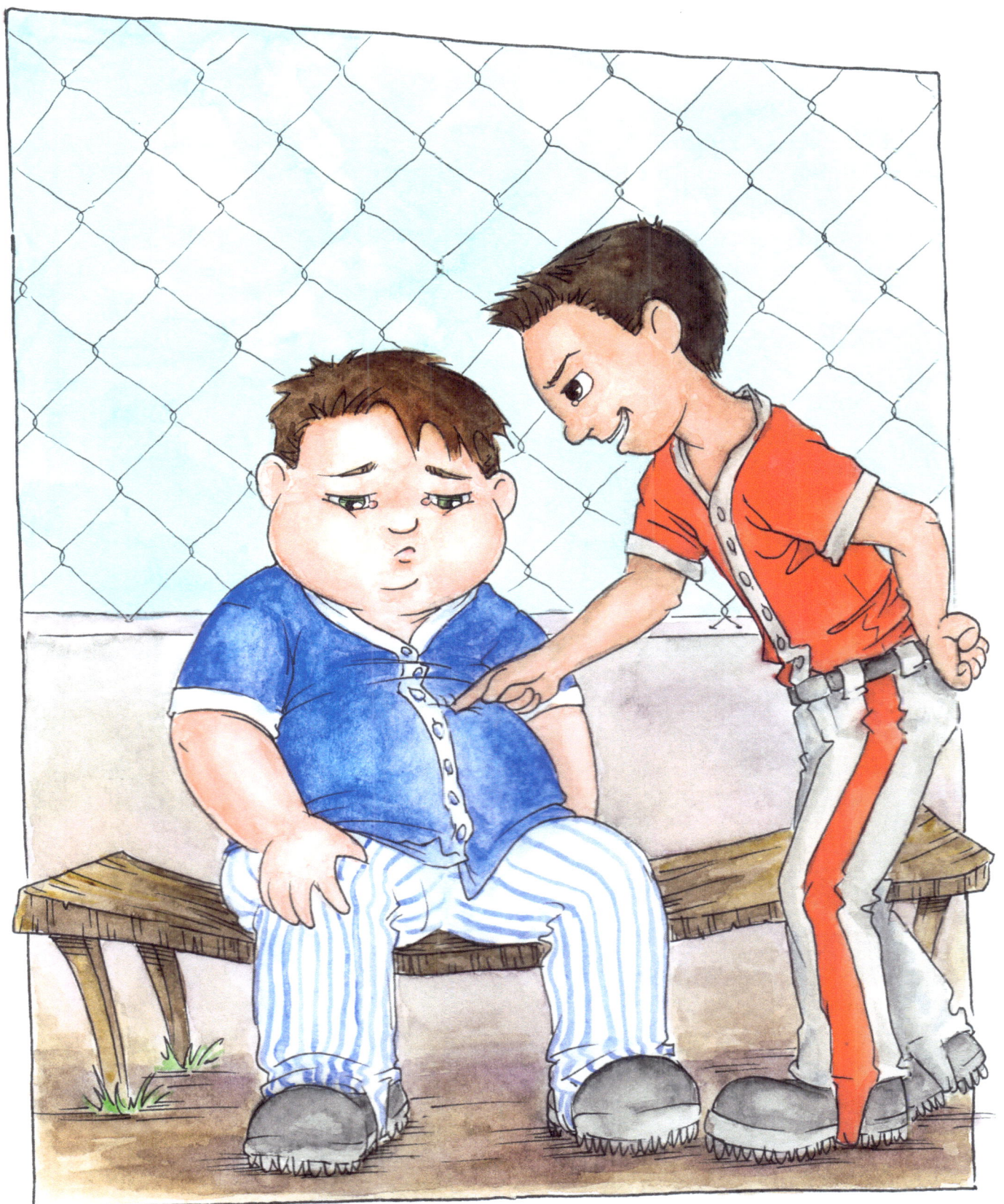

"Hey Peter, where are you?" called Sam and Mike. Peter sadly went to join his friends.

"What's wrong, Peter?" Mike asked him.

"It's Tony again. He called me...that name. I wanted to tell him to stop, but last time..."

"He's a big bully," Sam said.

Peter nodded. What am I going to do, guys? Tony and his friends are making me crazy! They act like I *want* to look like this!"

"It's time you showed Tony just what you are made of," Sam told him.

"He knows what I'm made of." Peter said. "I'm a fatty."

Mike told Peter, "It's your food choices that are fatty, Peter, not you. WE know what you really are – a great pitcher and a great friend."

"Yeah!" Sam said. "Let's get you in shape to pitch the next game against Tony's team. He will learn that it is not nice to push other people around."

Peter brightened. "Really? That's great. If we work together, I know I can do it!"

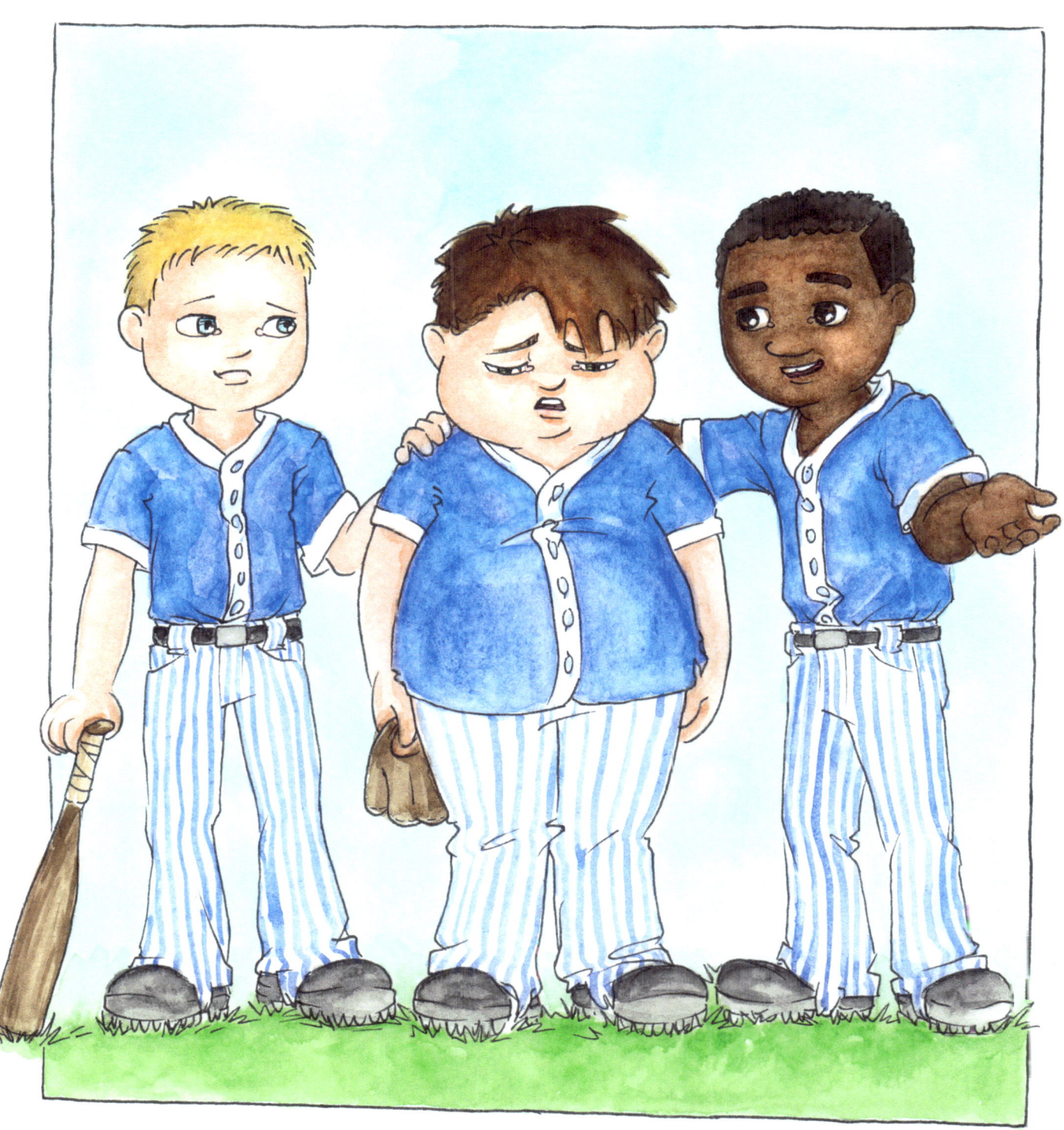

It was the next day, while the boys were eating breakfast together at school, when they decided to start Peter's new healthy eating habits. No more starchy pancakes, thick maple syrup, greasy bacon and artificially flavored strawberry milk. Instead, Sam and Mike put scrumptious scrambled eggs, whole wheat toast, orange juice and a shiny apple on Peter's tray.

During lunch, Tony strutted over to Peter, Sam, and Mike's table. "Hey Peter Pudgy, what's for lunch? The same old junk food!" Tony snickered and poked Peter with his finger.

Sam stood up next to Peter. "Just leave him alone."

Tony glared at the three boys. "I was leaving anyways. Losers."

Without a word, Peter threw out his fatty hot dog, oily potato chips, sugary cookies, and sickly sweet soda. Sam and Mike picked him out a better lunch: a whole wheat sandwich made with lean and tasty turkey, green leafy lettuce and tangy yellow mustard, along with fresh carrots, juicy grapes and low fat milk. Peter loved the tastes and the smells of the new foods he tried that day.

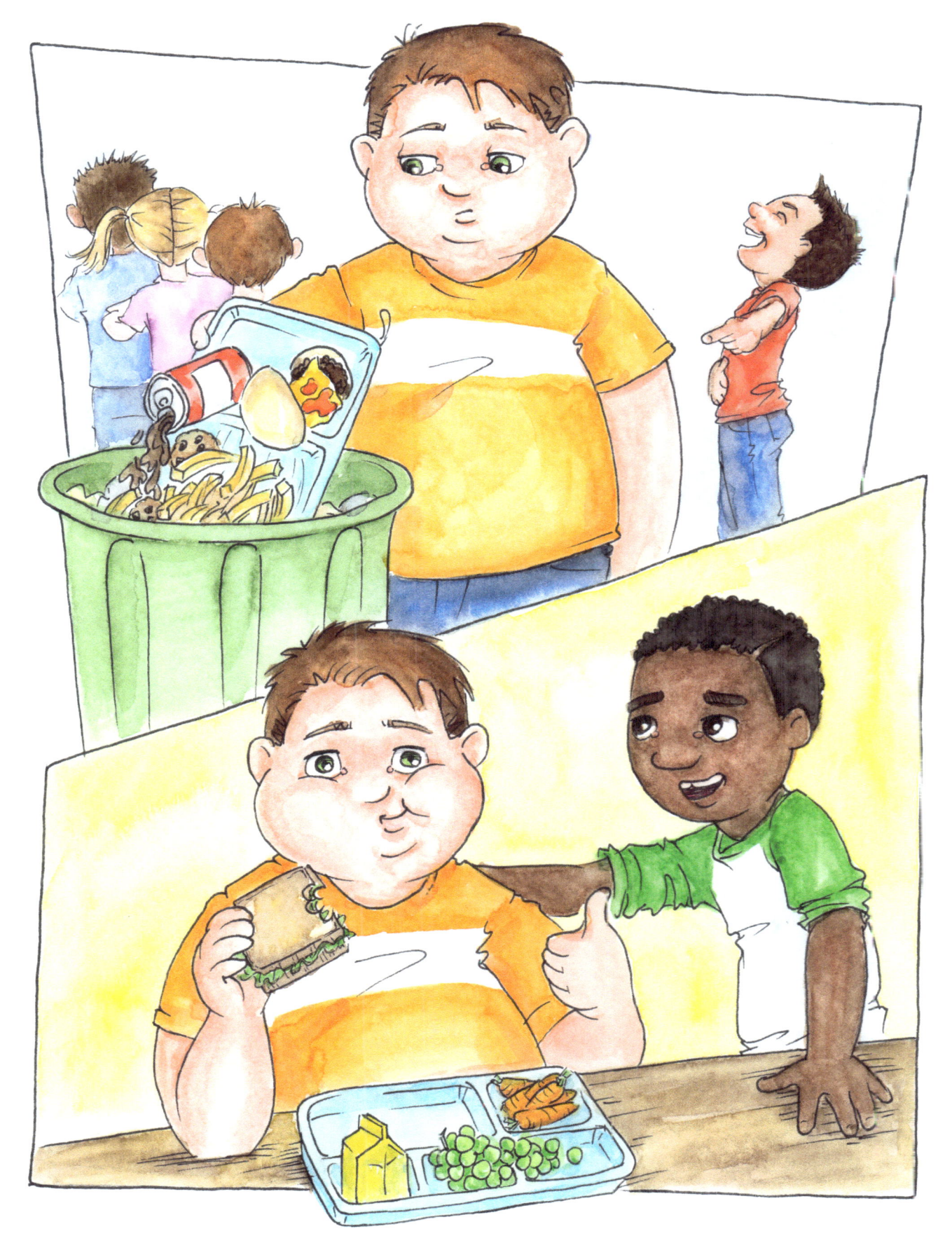

Weeks went by, and Peter was surprised how much he enjoyed eating healthy meals. One day, as Peter watered his Mother's garden, he thought about how he was losing weight. That was good, but he didn't feel much stronger or faster. How was he supposed to help his team win against Tony's team?

Suddenly the ground rumbled and up popped Crispy Carrot, Bella Broccoli and Tommy Tomato. They stretched their limbs, looked at Peter and thanked him for watering them and helping them grow.

Peter blinked his eyes, blinked again and asked, "Are you real?"

"Oh, we're real," Crispy Carrot tipped her green leaves and said, "My job is to give you vitamins that help your eyesight so you can see the baseball clearly. I'm crunchy, orange and hearty."

Bella Broccoli bowed, "I'm also full of vitamins and good things that make your body strong. I'm a lovely shade of green, bigger than a bean and very nutritious."

Tommy Tomato rolled around. "It's my turn. My job is to build your body up to fight germs and to keep you from getting sick. I'm red, round and yummy."

Peter looked at the three vegetables. "I can't believe it! Talking veggies!"

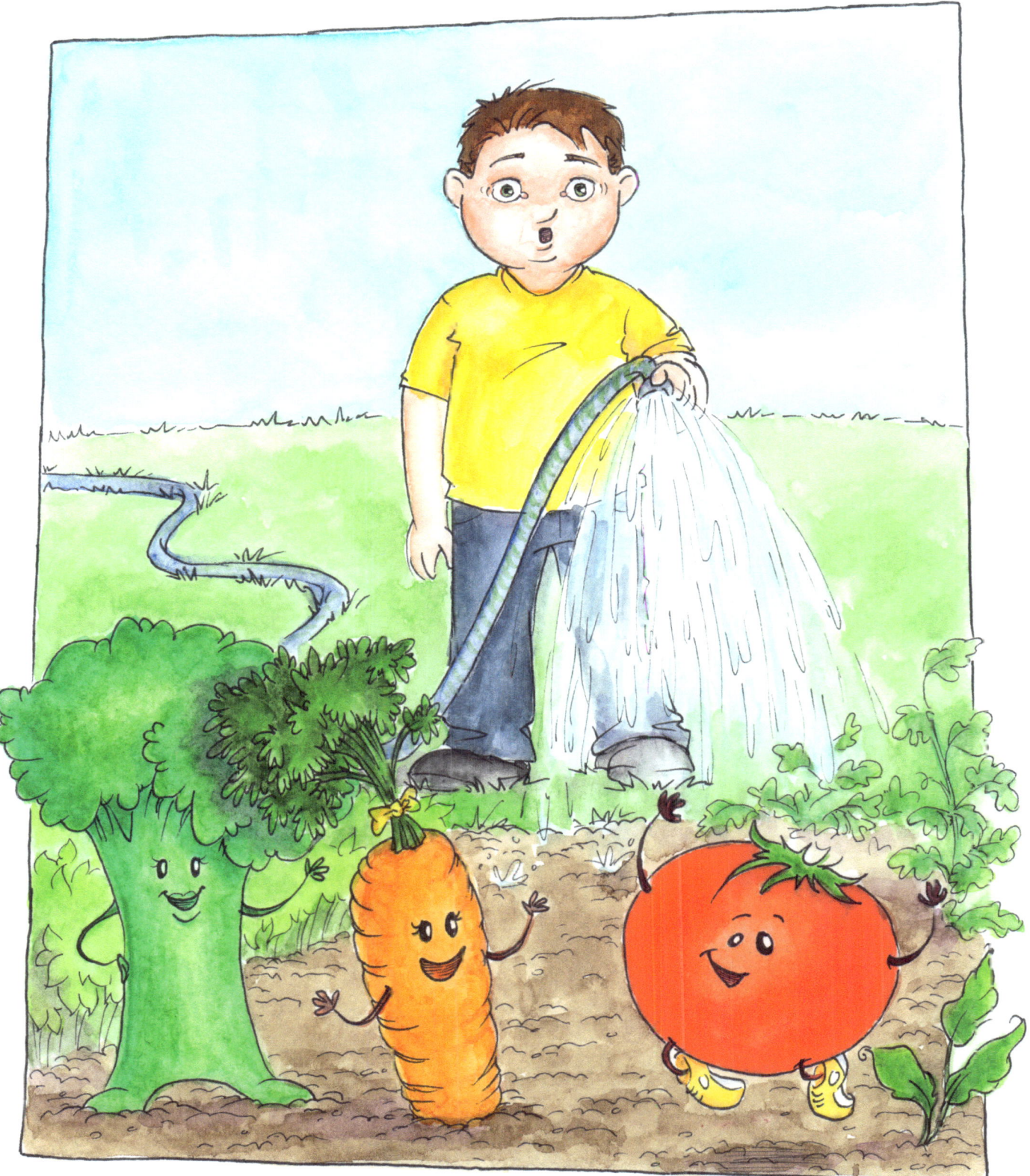

"We're here to help! What's your story?" Bella Broccoli asked.

Peter told them about Tony bullying him and how Sam and Mike were helping him eat better. "I know I'm losing weight because my pants are much looser and I have to wear a belt. But I'm not feeling stronger or faster. I'm not sure I'll ever be much help to my team."

"Peter, you have two great friends who have helped you make excellent food choices. Now let's do some exciting things to get your body moving! We'll help you get healthy nutrients so you can run faster and build bigger muscles." Crispy Carrot made a muscle with her carrot-arm and acted like she was lifting weights.

That afternoon, everyone met in Peter's backyard and came up with a plan. Crispy Carrot, Bella Broccoli and Tommy Tomato would make sure Peter ate healthy foods. Right away, Peter's new vegetable friends came up with delicious new recipes and taught the entire family how to cook low fat meals to help Peter build strong muscles and a strong body.

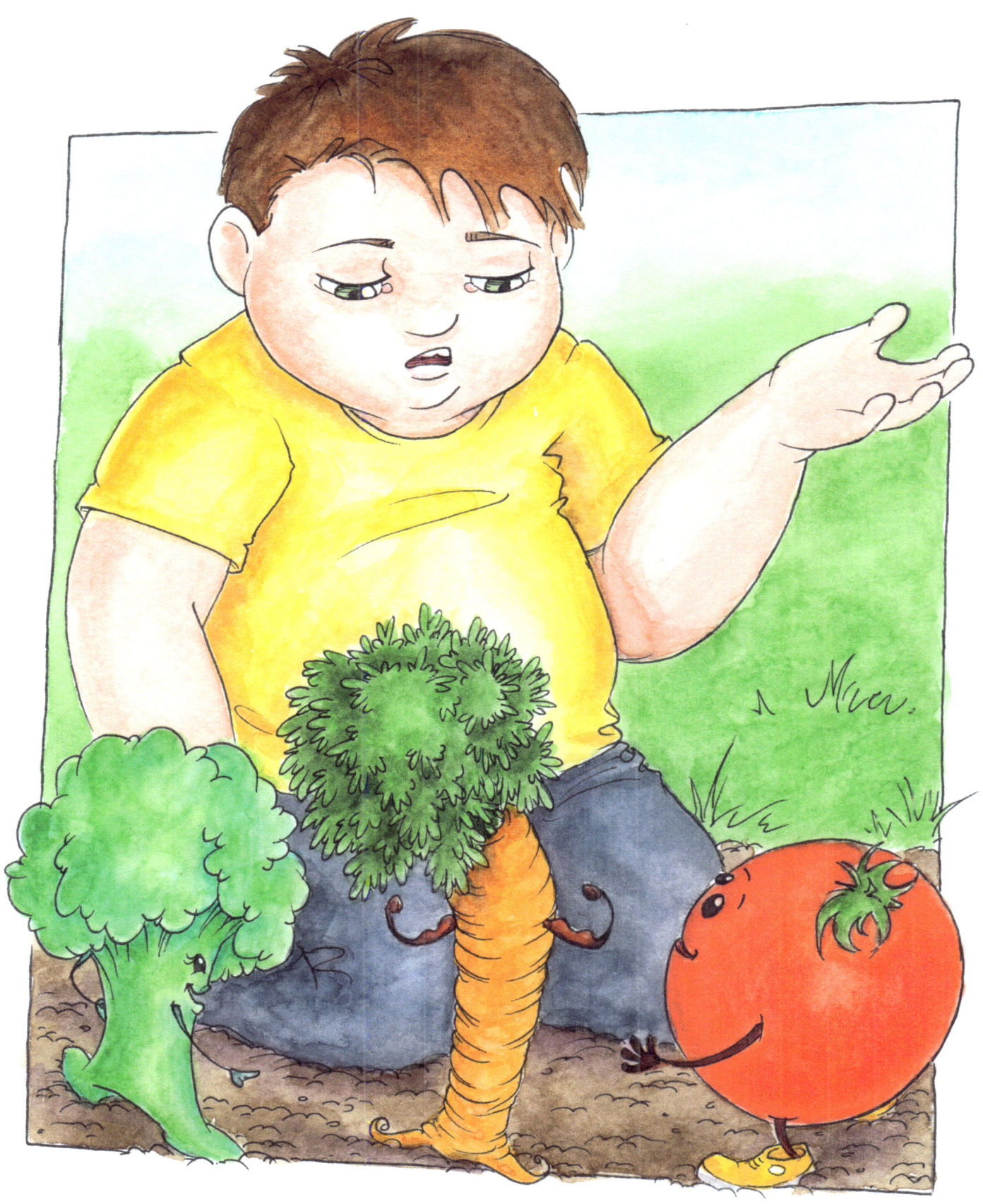

More weeks went by, and all the while Sam and Mike helped Peter get in shape. The three boys ran around the track, threw the ball around the bases, and played games with other kids. They rode their bikes, helped neighbors rake their lawns, and cleaned up their rooms. Peter had so much fun. He didn't play as many video games and spent more time outside. He didn't feel heavy or sad anymore. Now he felt happy and healthy and full of energy.

Every day, Peter pitched fast balls, sliders, and curve balls to Sam and Mike. At team practice, they ran bases, did speed drills and push-ups … and Peter did too! He worked hard and shared what he had learned about being healthy with his teammates. They all wanted to be ready for their game against the Crushers.

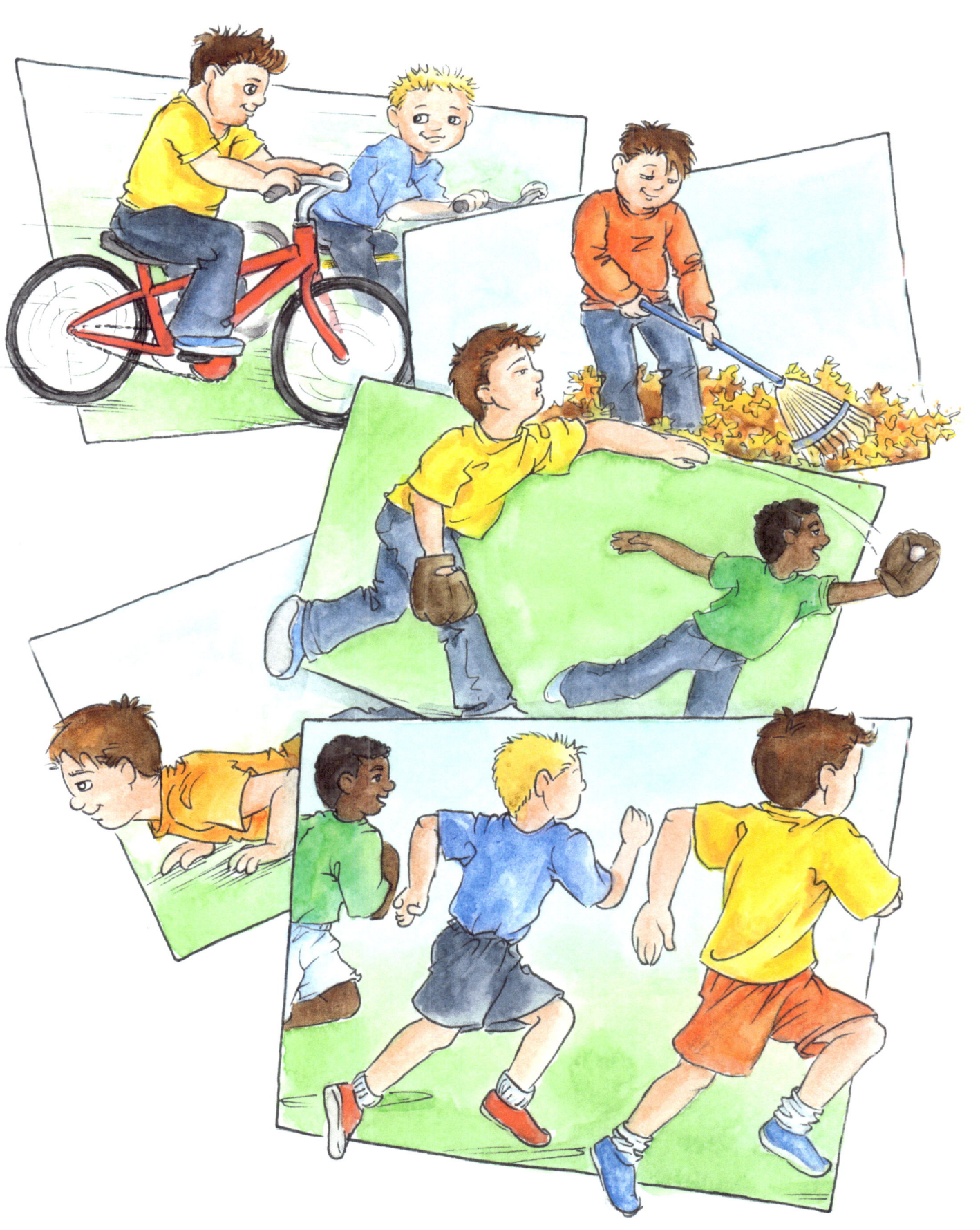

It was the day of the Big Game! Peter was so proud when Coach told him that he would be the starting pitcher. Peter had butterflies in his stomach as he stood on the pitcher's mound. He hoped he wouldn't let his team down.

Tony came up to bat. "Look, there's Peter Pudgy!" he taunted. "Ha! Ha! You're such a loser, Peter. Do you really think your puny arms can throw the ball this far? Ha, ha, ha!"

The rest of the Crushers started jeering, "Losers! Losers! Losers!"

Peter felt that old sad feeling coming back. But then ... *Wait a minute*, Peter thought, *I'm NOT a fatty anymore!*

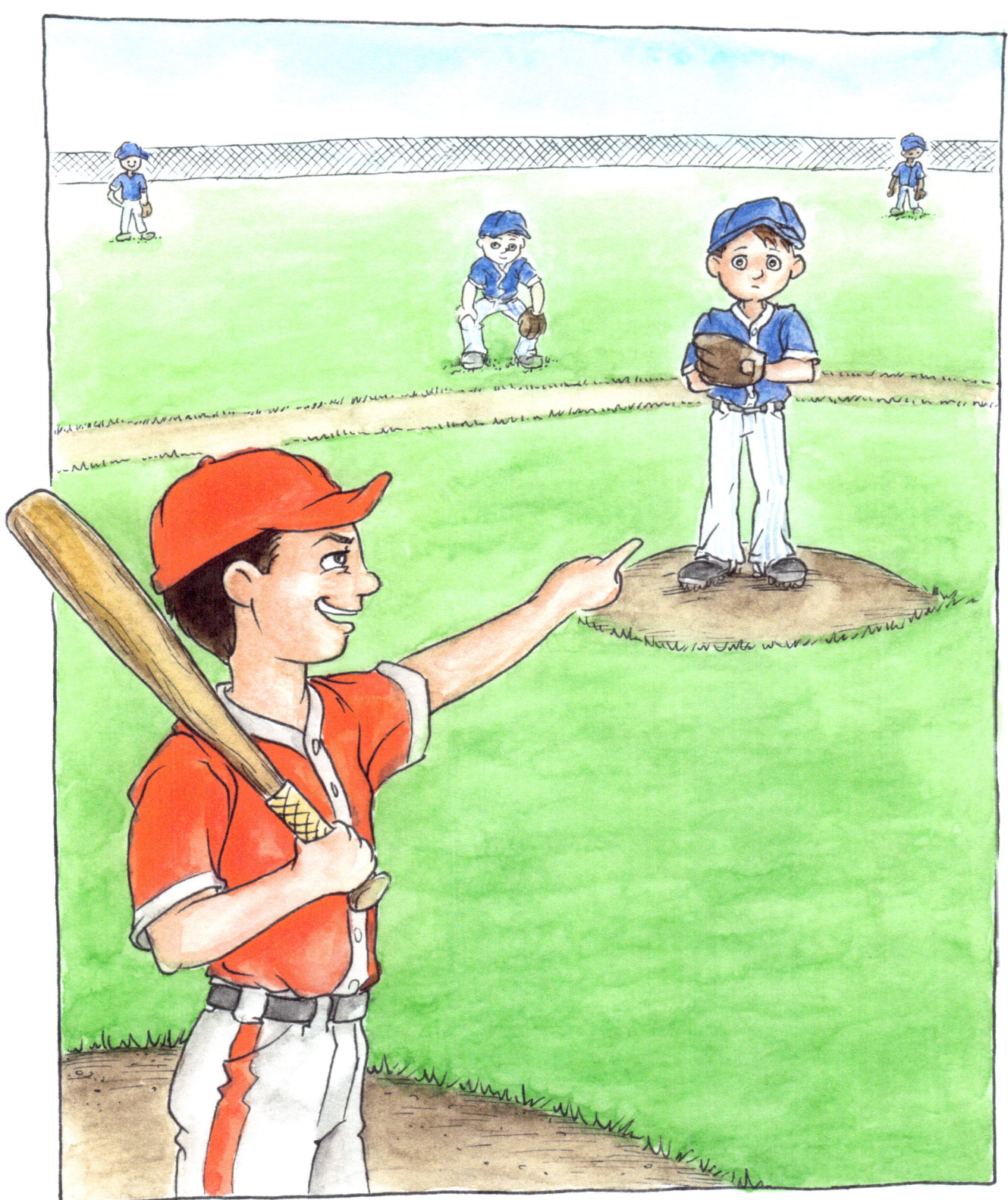

Peter threw his first pitch to Tony. The ball streaked right through the center of home plate. "Strike one!" the umpire said. Tony blinked.

Peter threw his second pitch. "Strike two!" said the umpire. Tony's mouth fell open in surprise. Peter was surprised too. He had never thrown the ball so fast before, and it was all because of his new and improved muscles.

Peter threw the third pitch. Tony swung with all his might ... and missed! "Strike three," called the umpire. "You're out!"

Tony was so shocked ... and *mad!* He stomped off to his bench, grumbling all the way. "You just wait until next time, Wimp!" He shook his fist at Peter.

His teammates joined in, taunting the Good Guys. "Losers! Losers! You can't beat *us!* Go home to your mommies—get back on the bus!"

"Don't listen to them, guys!" Peter encouraged his team. "We *can* win!"

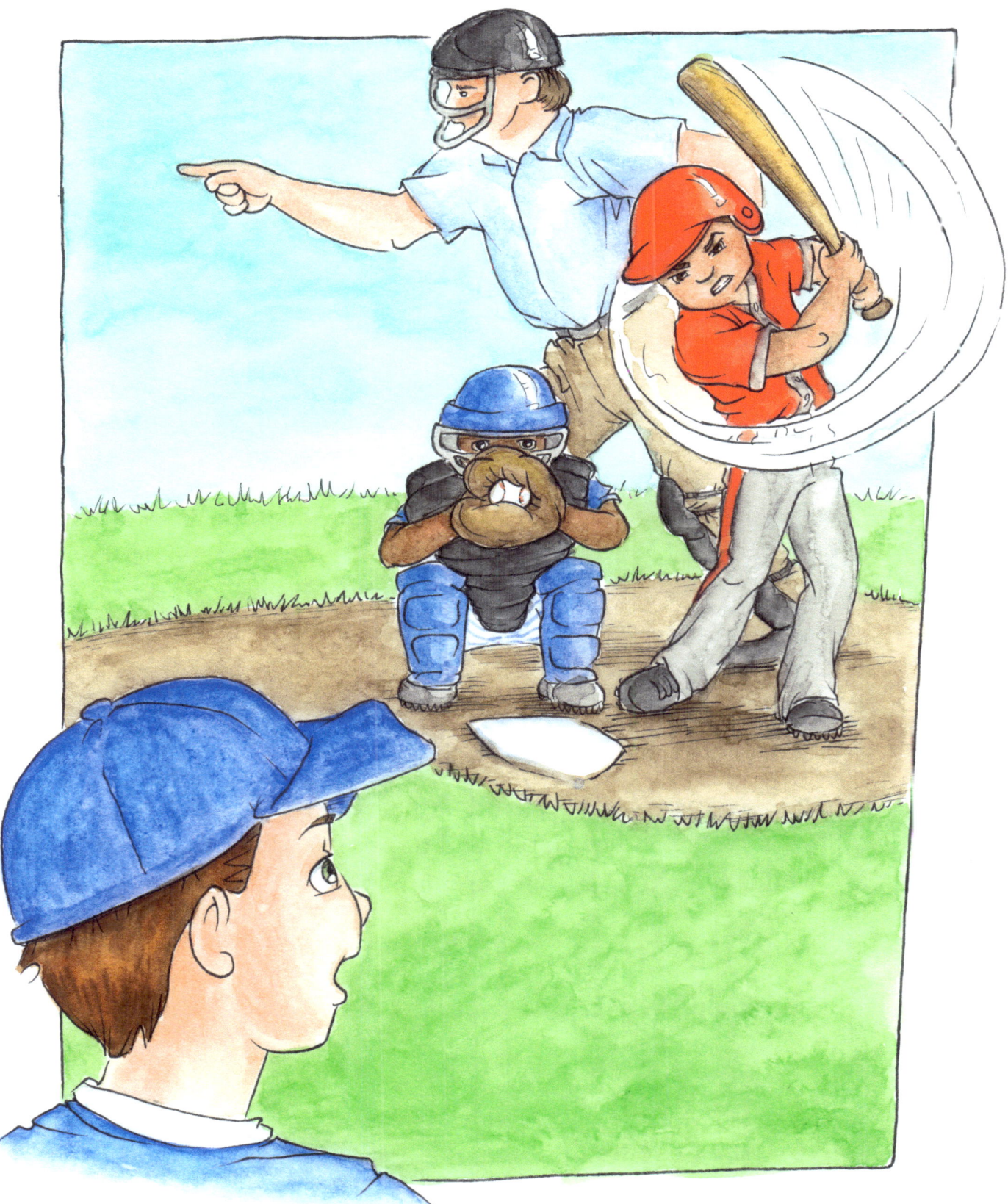

And they *did* win!

At the end of the ninth inning, the Good Guys had five runs and the Crushers had scored three. There were three men on base and two outs. Tony came up to bat. Peter's heart beat faster but he thought, *I can do this! I can do this!* He threw the first pitch. Strike one! He threw the second pitch. Strike two! He threw the third pitch. Strike three! He had struck Tony out. They had won the game!

All the Good Guys jumped up and down, throwing their hats and gloves into the air in celebration. They rushed to the pitcher's mound, chanting "Peter! Peter! Peter!" Everyone slapped him on the back, giving high fives, and carried him off the field on their shoulders. Looking up to the stands, Peter saw his family standing and waving. Peter felt so happy he thought he might explode!

Coach walked up to Peter, and with a big smile, said "Peter, you are such a good example and a great leader for the team. How would you like to be our captain?"

The Good Guys cheered, "Hooray, Peter! Hooray!"

All Peter could do was grin from ear to ear. His dream had come true!

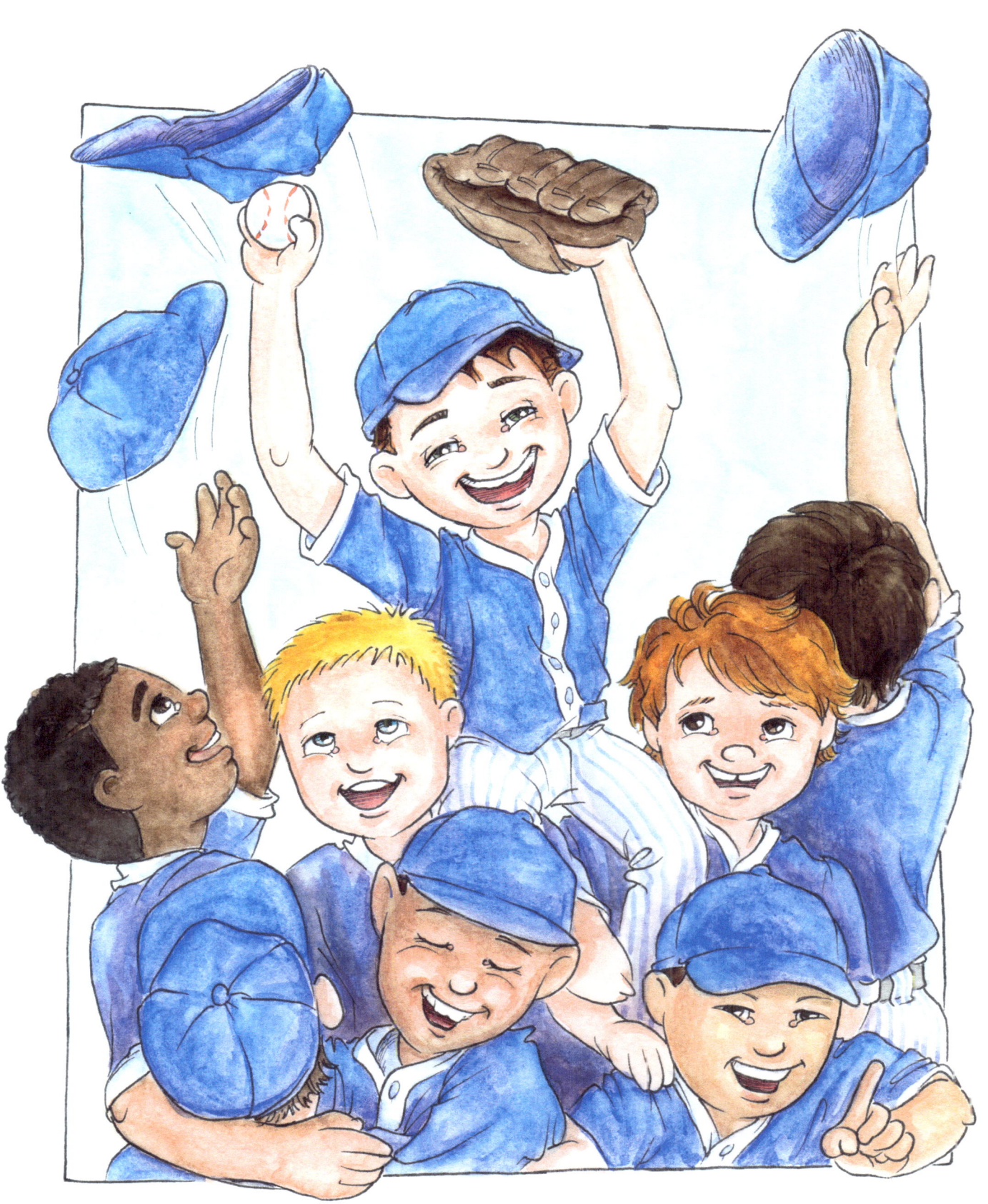

The Veggie Friends popped up. "Congratulations!" Bella Broccoli said.

"We are so proud of you," Tommy Tomato said, rolling over to playfully bump Peter's leg. "You did it! You are the captain of the Good Guys!"

"Yes," said Crispy Carrot. "You tried new foods, different exercises, and you didn't give up! You became a great role model for other kids!"

"No more Peter Pudgy!" Bella Broccoli smiled at him. "You are now Peter Proud!"

Peter laughed. "Yes, I am, and it feels great! I'm not going to be Peter Pudgy, ever again!"

The Veggie Friends began to march away.

"Wait!" Peter called. "Where are you going?"

"Off to see if we can find another boy or girl we can help, just like you." Crispy Carrot said.

Tommy Tomato nodded. "Yes, sir! There are lots of kids out there who need to learn about better ways to eat and become active, healthy children."

"Thank you so much! I'll never forget what you've done for me." Peter waved goodbye to his Veggie Friends.

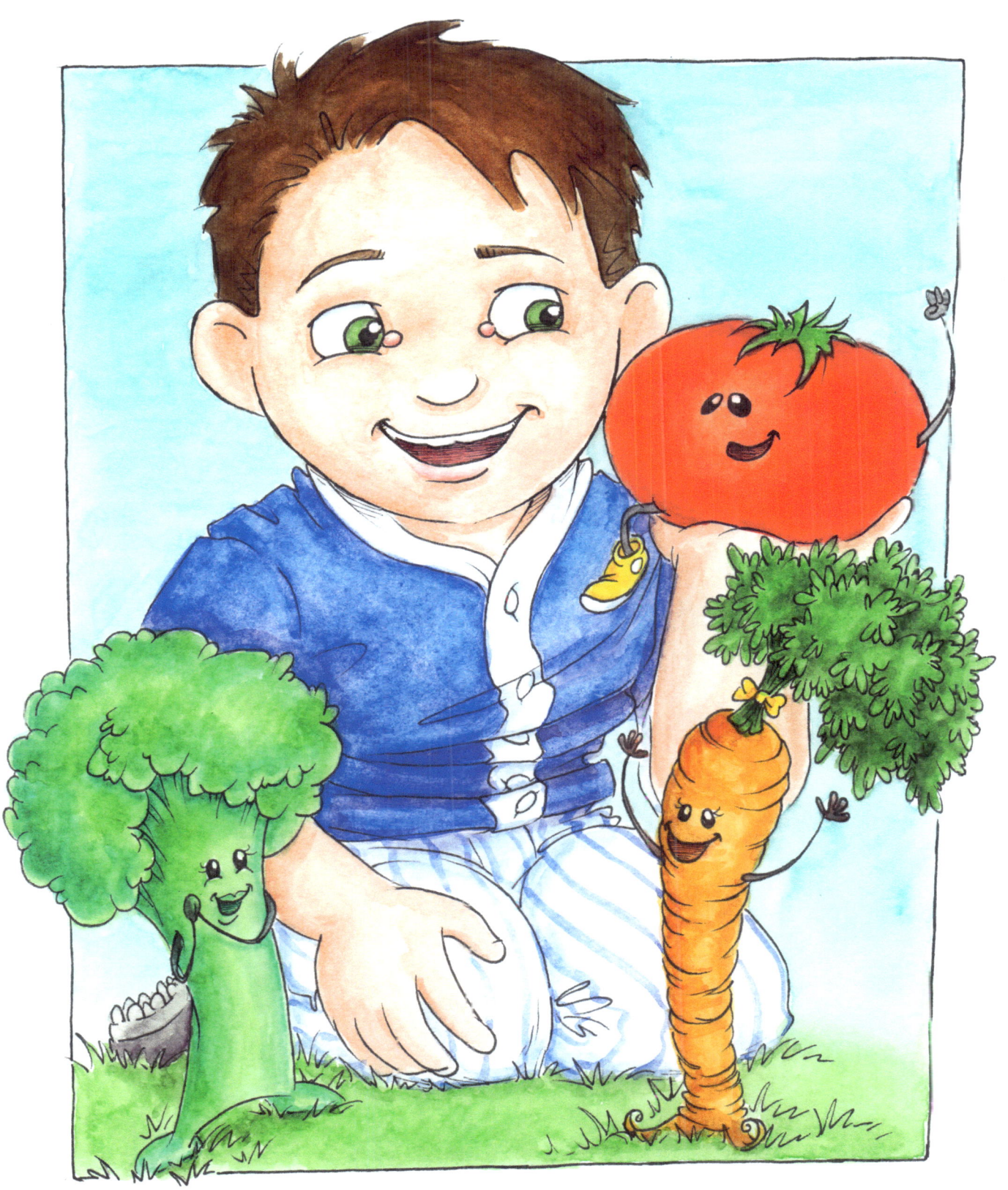

As everyone left the field to go home, Sam and Mike caught up with Peter. "Way to go, Captain!" Mike said. "You did awesome. You saved the game!"

"Yeah," said Sam, "we knew you could do it! You are our hero!"

"Aw, thanks, guys," Peter replied. "We're all heroes. I couldn't have done this without you."

Sam threw his arm around Peter. "From now on, we'll be three great baseball players."

Mike put his arm around Peter's other shoulder. "Three best friends!"

"Three *healthy* heroes!" said Peter.

And that is how Peter Pudgy became Peter Proud.

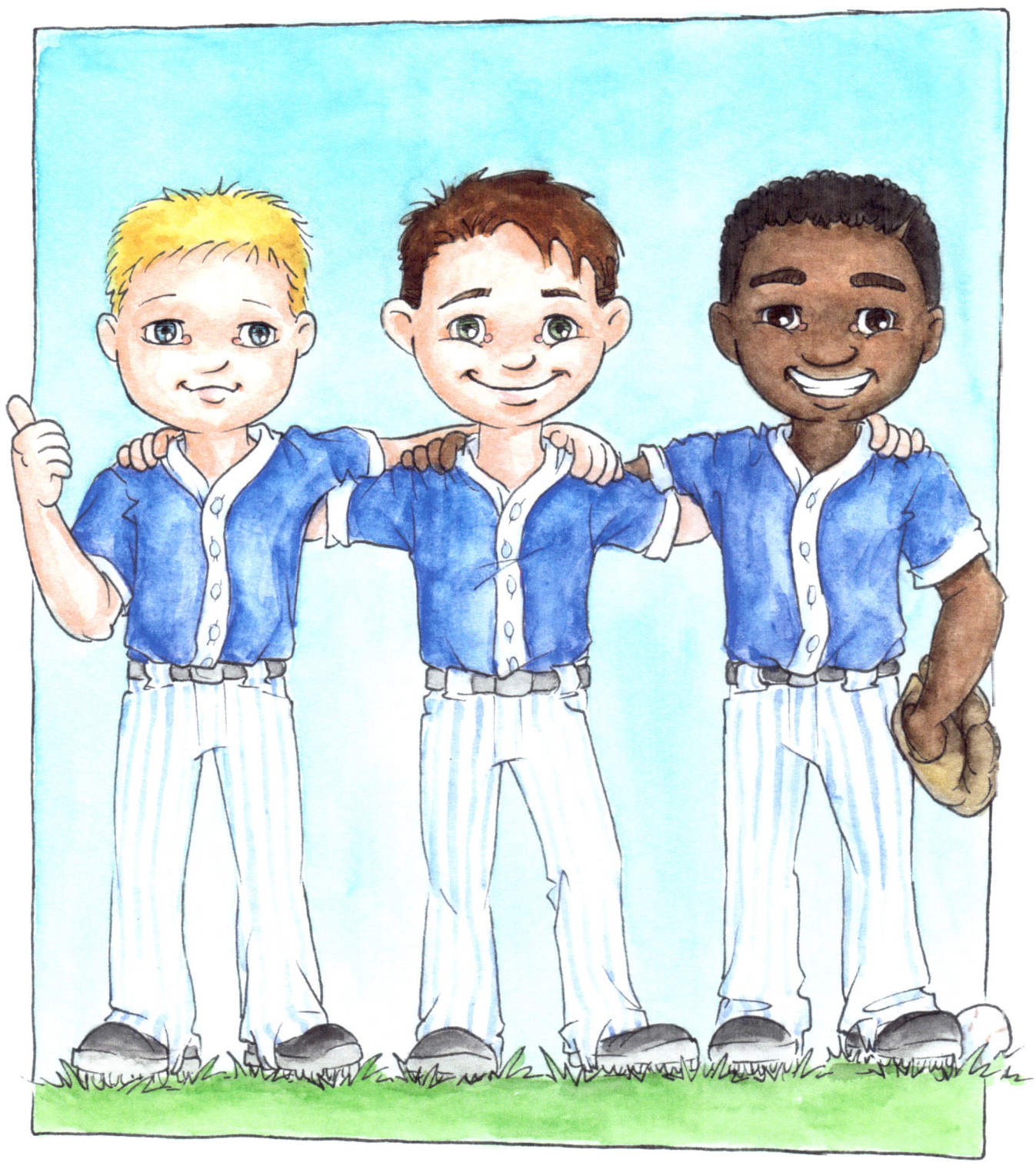

www.ingramcontent.com/pod-product-compliance
Lightning Source LLC
Chambersburg PA
CBHW060819290526
45792CB00005BB/1721